I0414714

PRAISE FOR GETTING A GOOD NIGHT'S SLEEP:
A PROBLEM-SOLVING SKILLS GUIDE

"For the last few years, I have known sleep is an area I should improve and have started to explore the science behind sleep to build my knowledge in this area. What I really like about this book, "Getting a Good Night's Sleep: A Problem Solving Skills Guide" is that it is a practical and pragmatic book that offers helpful advice but also tools to embrace and actually hold me accountable. There are no excuses anymore-if I really place an importance on getting those-7-9 hours sleep each night then I actually can make that happen through the format of this valuable book and the templates included. Thank you for making it possible!"

Katrina Bromell,

360° Coach, Regional Director of Life in Balance Careers, Australia

"Focusing on sleep may appear like giving attention to a lazy man's hobby. Dr Adrian Low and Dr Patrick Gwyer have given sleep its dignity back and for our own good. This mini book is a resource that will help you live a healthy life."

Dr Margaret Kagwe, PhD,

Esteem Psychology Magazine

"How can you cope with insomnia? I will advise you 3 key solutions, firstly Prayer, secondly this book and thirdly a good psychologist like Dr Adrian Low."

Raymond Fu,

CEO, LOGOS Group of Companies

Getting a good night's sleep:

A problem-solving skills guide

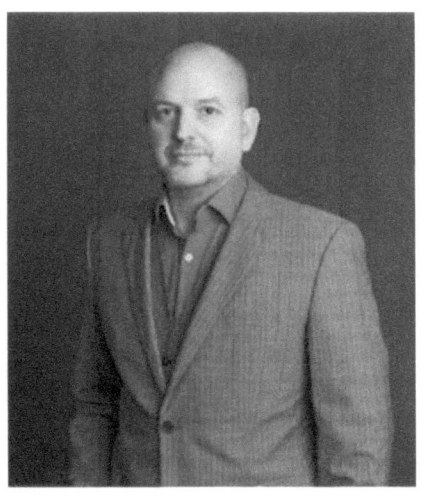

Dr Patrick Gwyer is registered with the United Kingdom's Health and Care Professions Council (HCPC), the British Psychology Society (BPS) and he is on the BPS Register of Applied Psychology Practice Supervisors. Dr Gwyer achieved the title Associate Fellow of the British Psychology Society (AFBPsS) and more recently was granted the status of Chartered Scientist (CSci). You can visit his website at www.DrPatrickGwyer.com

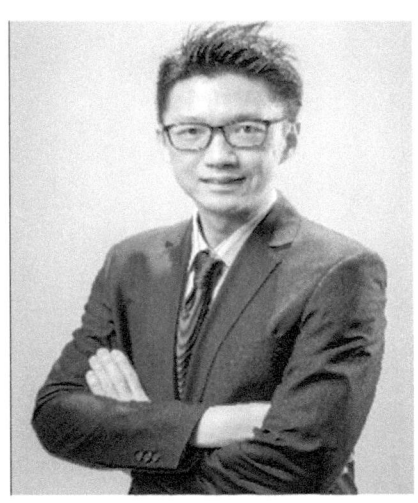

Dr Adrian Low is a chartered psychologist (BPS) that has graduated with a Doctor of Clinical & Industrial/Organisational Psychology from California Southern University in the USA. He also holds a master's degree in Education from The Chinese University of Hong Kong.

Dr Low's workplace stress research has won the presidential award for doctoral research excellence at the California Southern University and since then he has been invited to be a keynote speaker in many conferences worldwide. Dr Low is the president of the Hong Kong Association of Psychology. Besides that, he is an adjunct faculty member at the University of Worcester as well as an adjunct lecturer at the HKU (university of Hong Kong) School of Professional and Continuing Education and the Hong Kong Polytechnic University. You can visit his website at www.DrAdrianLow.com

Dedicated to

All the insomniacs and to anyone who is suffering

from any form of mental illness...

Getting a good night's sleep:
A problem-solving skills guide

Dr Pat Gwyer PhD DClinPsych MSc

Associate Fellow of the British Psychological Society

Chartered Psychologist

Clinical Psychologist

Chartered Scientist

And

Dr Adrian Low PsyD, CPsychol

Chartered Psychologist of the British Psychological Society,

President of the Hong Kong Association of Psychology

TABLE OF CONTENTS

Disclaimer

Although the authors and publisher have made every effort to ensure that the information contained in this ebook was correct at the time of publication, the authors and the publisher do not assume and hereby disclaim any liability to any party for loss, damage, or disruption caused by any omissions or errors resulting from accident, negligence or any other cause.

The information contained in the ebook is intended to increase your awareness of some factors that might be connected to your quality of sleep. This is intended to make you more informed about your sleep and what you may be able to do to improve it. It is presented as general advice on this area and is not intended as a substitute or replacement for the advice of any relevantly trained, qualified, licenced and registered mental or physical health practitioner.

The reader should consult such a professional in matters relating to their sleep and health and wellbeing, especially with regards the diagnosis of any medical symptoms, their use of medication, or other therapeutic approaches they may require.

INTRODUCTION

Evidence has shown that sleep is key to your wellbeing and that without restful sleep, physical and mental wellness and wellbeing suffers.

Unfortunately, when life gets hectic, getting a good night's sleep—when it is, in fact, the most needed - becomes increasingly difficult. Poor sleep can include any of the following.

    i.   Not being able to fall asleep
   ii.   Not getting restful sleep
  iii.   Early waking

However, there are many things you can do to help get a better night's sleep. Before we look at the things, we can do let's just look into sleep in a little more detail.

WHY SLEEP IS IMPORTANT

Sleep has a restorative effect on our bodies and minds and is essential to our wellbeing, health and our ability to function. As well as helping us recover from our day's activity, it also prepares and refreshes us for the next day.

Sleep is so important it is not an option or luxury, but an essential. Without sleep we more easily become confused, disoriented, find concentration and decision making harder, have problems with our memory, make more mistakes, decrease our motivation and problem-solving ability and find our emotions harder to manage. A lack of sleep reduces our resilience and our ability to deal with psychological stress.

Our physical health also suffers when we do not get enough sleep, and lack of sleep is associated with weight gain (you eat more sugary and fatty foods to give you energy). In addition, a lack of sleep has been shown to be linked to high blood pressure, heart disease, obesity, diabetes and our immune system's ability to work effectively.

Evidence has shown that almost 20% of accidents on major roads are sleep-related and that sleep-related accidents are more likely to result in a fatality or serious injury. In addition, when people don't get enough sleep, they are more likely to have workplace accidents

Benefits of sleep

As we as the detrimental effects of a lack of sleep, there are also a number of benefits to getting a good night's sleep. These include improving;

- Creativity, vitality and productivity
- Life expectancy
- Attention, memory, concentration, and problem-solving ability
- Ability to manage stress and resilience
- Physical health
- Improves social intelligence

Part of the solid back four

There are four interconnect basics needed for wellbeing. These include a healthy diet (and hydration), physical activity, a routine and sleep.

Sleep is a very important basic and getting a good night's sleep should become one of your wellbeing habits. Getting a good night's sleep is an essential, not a negotiable or a luxury.

Two common myths about sleep

"A few hours of missing sleep won't hurt."

Even losing one hour of sleep can affect your ability to think and respond and impact your immune system.

"I can catch up on my sleep later or stock it up for when needed."

Although catching up on lost sleep is helpful and can go towards relieving your "sleep debt", it will not completely make up for the lack of sleep.

Think of a car engine that has continuously been run without a break. A later service might help, but some damage to the engine will have occurred. Sleeping later also has a knock-on effect and make it much harder to go to sleep the following nights and get up the following morning. It is not possible to stock up on sleep.

How much sleep do I need?

There is a difference between the amount of sleep necessary to "get by" and the amount required to function at your best. Due to the demands of modern day life, people now are typically getting enough sleep to get by, rather than what they need to be at their best.

Many people report that they "get by" with six to seven hours of sleep a night, which although they think is good, is actually not likely to be enough. Often people think that they are too busy, life too hectic, and they have too much to do to "waste it" sleeping. However, this is a false economy. We are much more productive and effective when we are rested and when sleep deprived we make more mistakes find concentrating harder so our performance and getting all those things done, actually decreases.

How much sleep we need, varies from person to person. Most healthy adults need between 7 to 9 hours of sleep per night to function at their best. This increases when we are mentally and physically busy and for children and teens who need even more.

Am I getting enough sleep?

The best way to see if you're getting enough sleep is to keep a diary of how many hours sleep you think you are getting (do this by recording the time you go to bed and get up each day) and compare that to how you are feeling throughout the day. If you're getting enough sleep, you'll feel energetic and alert all day long. If you are not getting enough sleep as well has having less energy and being less alert, you may experience one or more of the things listed below. Go through the list and tick the ones you feel apply to you.

SIGNS YOU AREN'T GETTING ENOUGH SLEEP

Sign you might not be getting enough sleep Tick those that apply to you	
Feeling drowsy during the day	
Feeling tired with no energy	
Craving sugary and fatty foods	
Experiencing "microsleeps" (brief episodes of sleep that happen while being awake)	
Using lots of caffeinate drinks to stay awake	
Falling asleep within a few minutes sitting down on the sofa or watching TV	
Lack of concentration, poor memory, difficulty with problem-solving, less creative	
Finding things harder to deal with, less resilient	
Being irritable and snappy for no reason	
Low mood, increased worry	
More aches & pains slower than usual recovery from illness or injury frequent colds & infections	
Relationship difficulties and reduced sex drive	
More clumsy, careless and accident prone	
Falling asleep within a few minutes of lying down in bed	
Needing an alarm clock to wake up on time	
Frequently oversleeping	
Have a hard time getting out of bed in the morning	
Feeling the need to sleep in on weekends	
Feeling like you don't get enough sleep	

Are there any other signs that you have noticed?

_____

_____

_____

_____

_____

_____

_____

_____

_____

Keeping a sleep diary can also help with increasing your understanding of your sleeping habits. The information you collect can also help you talk to your GP about your difficulties and help them make a possible diagnosis.

Keeping a sleep diary also makes you more proactive in managing your sleep. From your diary, you will be able to understand more precisely what is going on, what thing you can try and how effective they are.

For example, you might notice that each time you drank alcohol before bedtime, while you might have fallen sleep quicker, you, however, awoke more frequently and felt unrefreshed in the morning. Or you might notice that certain things, like being active or not napping during the day, lead to better sleep.

When you keep a sleep diary, you are better able to notice what is helpful and unhelpful to your sleep. From this, you find ways you can increase the helpful and decrease the unhelpful.

When improving your sleep think of it as a problem to be solved. The problem you wish to address is that the quality and quantity of sleep is not sufficient for your wellbeing.

Using the information in this ebook, and what you have collected from your sleep diary, try different things until you can improve the quality and quantity of your sleep and have solved your sleep problem.

SLEEP DIARY

Complete the diary each morning. "Day 1" is the morning you begin. Do not worry too much about giving exact answers, a best "guestimate" will do.

Sleep diary	Mon	Tues	Weds	Thurs	Fri	Sat	Sun
What time did you go to bed last night?							
How long did it take you to fall asleep?							
How many times did you wake during the night?							
When (if) you woke during the night, in total for how long do you think you were awake for?							
What time did you finally wake up?							
What time did you get up?							
How long did you spend in bed last night (from first getting in, to finally getting up)							
Did you struggle to wake up when it was time to get up?	Yes/ No	Yes/ No	Yes/ No	Yes/ No	Yes/ No	Yes/ No	Yes/ No
How would you rate the quality of the sleep you got? (1 is low, and 10 is high)							
Did you feel refreshed when you woke up?	Yes/ No	Yes/ No	Yes/ No	Yes/ No	Yes/ No	Yes/ No	Yes/ No
What it easy or difficult to fall asleep?	Easy/ Difficult	Easy/ Difficult	Easy/ Difficult	Easy/ Difficult	Easy/ Difficult	Easy/ Difficult	Easy/ Difficult
What disturbed your sleep? physical aches or pains psychological or emotional worries, e.g. stress, worry environmental, e.g. noise, lights, comfort							

WHAT INTERFERES WITH A GOOD NIGHT'S SLEEP

Often there is a "vicious cycle" between lack of sleep, the factors that cause a lack of sleep and the symptoms of a lack of sleep. For example, a lack of sleep has been shown to increase depression and anxiety.

When we experience depression or anxiety, we often have racing thoughts and powerful and different to manage emotions. These then lead to further problems with sleep because we lie awake at night worrying. When we know this, we can address sleep problems indirectly and directly by breaking the vicious cycle associated with poor sleep and by doing things to improve our sleep skills.

If you are having trouble sleeping, and you lie awake at night worrying about your inability to sleep, notice these thoughts and the emotions they create and mindfully let them go. Funny as it might sound, people often lie awake at night thinking and worrying about the fact that they are not sleeping. As a result, their thoughts and worries about not sleeping end up being the thing that keeps them awake!

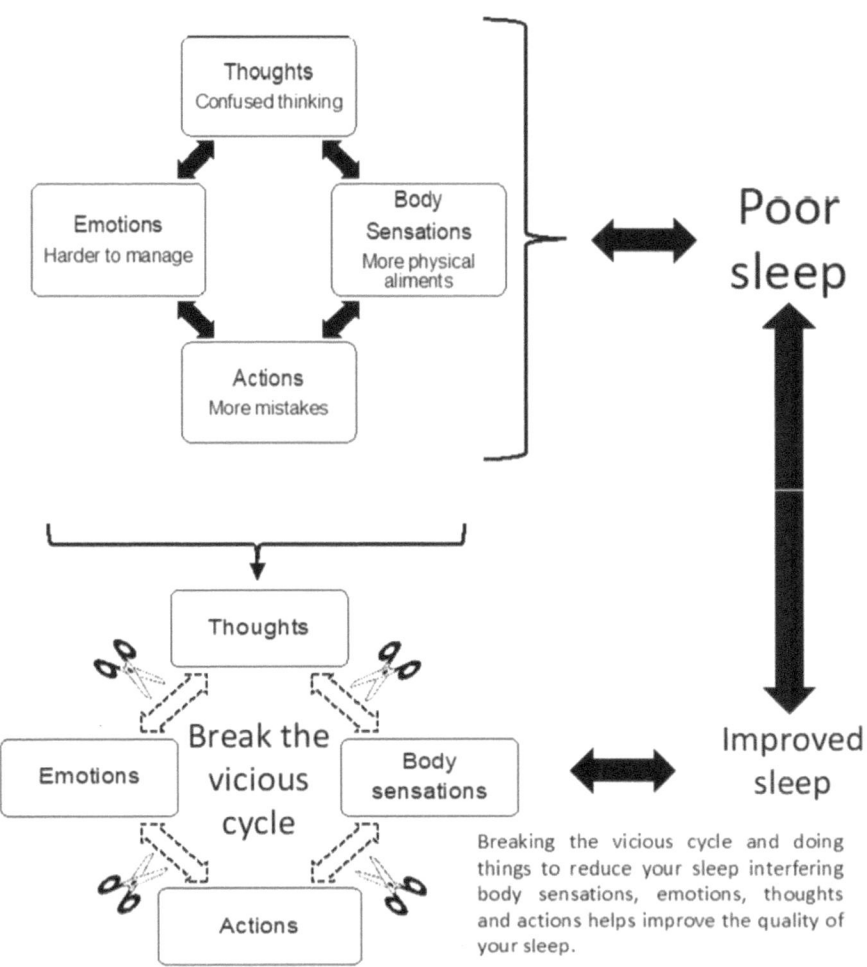

Figure 1: Break the vicious cycle and improve sleep skills

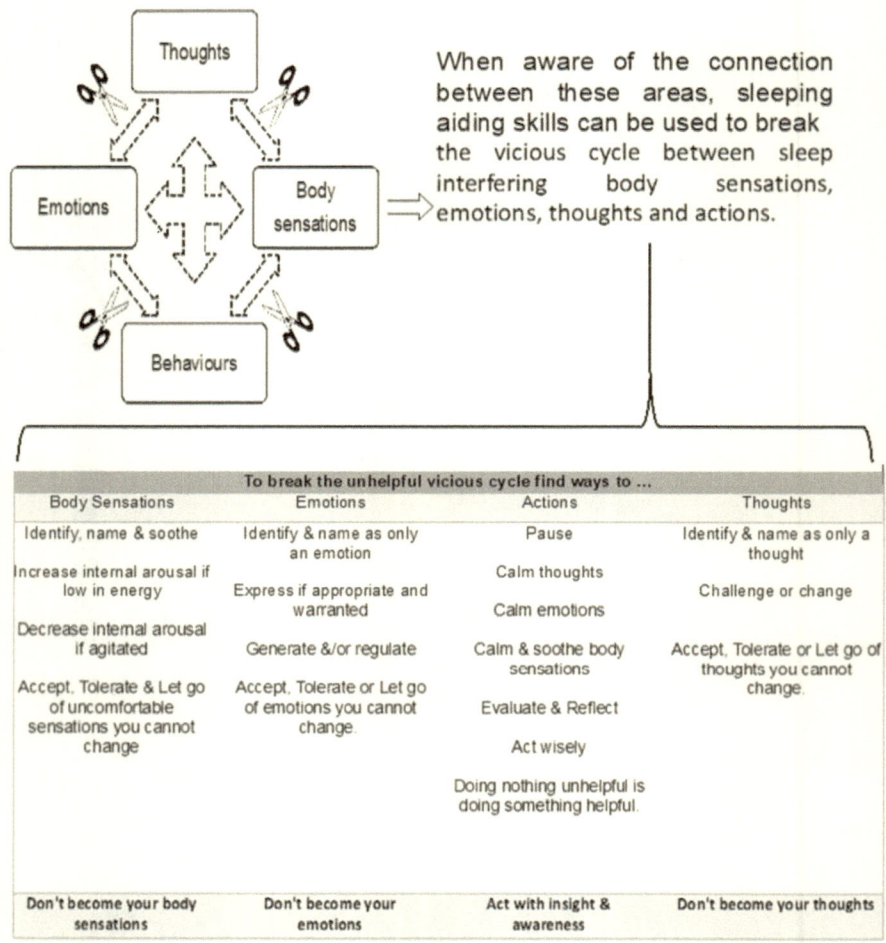

When aware of the connection between these areas, sleeping aiding skills can be used to break the vicious cycle between sleep interfering body sensations, emotions, thoughts and actions.

To break the unhelpful vicious cycle find ways to ...			
Body Sensations	Emotions	Actions	Thoughts
Identify, name & soothe	Identify & name as only an emotion	Pause	Identify & name as only a thought
Increase internal arousal if low in energy		Calm thoughts	
	Express if appropriate and warranted	Calm emotions	Challenge or change
Decrease internal arousal if agitated	Generate &/or regulate	Calm & soothe body sensations	
Accept, Tolerate & Let go of uncomfortable sensations you cannot change	Accept, Tolerate or Let go of emotions you cannot change.	Evaluate & Reflect	Accept, Tolerate or Let go of thoughts you cannot change.
		Act wisely	
		Doing nothing unhelpful is doing something helpful.	
Don't become your body sensations	Don't become your emotions	Act with insight & awareness	Don't become your thoughts

Figure 2: Break the vicious cycle and improve sleep skills[1]

---

[1] See the stress busting course for more details on this

SOME SLEEP SKILLS THAT WILL HELP YOU GET A BETTER NIGHT'S SLEEP

- Exercise and be active and avoid napping during the day so that you are physically tired at night.

- Eat a light snack before going to bed or drink a glass of milk. Make sure you don't eat heavy, fatty foods or eat and drink so much that you feel bloated and full, as this will make getting to sleep much harder.

- If you're in bed and can't sleep, DON'T turn on the television or electronic devices, or turn on bright lights. Notice you cant sleep, do not make a judgment about this or predictions about how you will feel. Take some deep breathes and relax your muscles.

- Be mindful of your thoughts and emotions; let go of any thoughts about sleep, let go of emotions that interfere with your getting to sleep and let your body relax.

- Just as you would do for a young child, establish a routine and bedtime ritual so that your body and mind can prepare for going to sleep. Getting up and going to bed at the same time every day, even on weekends, can help with this.

- Avoid alcohol, nicotine and caffeine before going to bed.

- Use your bed only for sleeping and only sleep when you are sleepy.

- Ensure that your bedroom is cool and quiet, that there is proper air circulation and that your bedding is comfortable.

- If you are on medication, check your medication's side effects.
- If you can't sleep, being mindful and doing muscle relaxation techniques will help relax you.

Getting your sleep under control takes time and effort, so it's essential that you don't give up. Trying these ten strategies should help you get a more restful night's sleep. Some may help more than others, and you may not need to do them all. However, with practice and effort, you will be able to improve the quality of sleep you get each night.

Other strategies you could use:

_____

_____

_____

_____

_____

_____

_____

_____

_____

_____

_____

What interferes with your sleep and what could you do to reduce this?

Things that interfere with my sleep	What I can do about this

IMPROVING SLEEP THROUGH MINDFULNESS, BREATHING, RELAXATION, GUIDED IMAGERY, AROMATHERAPY

Sleep aiding activities

Mindful body scan

(you can also use this with the progressive muscle relaxation exercise)

To do this mindfulness activity, complete the following steps. As you do each step, be curious and interested in what you notice but don't make judgements. Decide upon a strategy at which point you will move your attention to the next body part. This may be after a set number of breaths; just make sure each body part receives attention during the inhalation and exhalation of your breath.

When your mind wonders, use bare attention to notice where it has wandered off to and then gently bring your attention back to the activity. You will be using constrictive mindful awareness to focus on the specific parts of your body and widespread awareness to focus on your whole body as well as how the pieces connect.

Importantly, notice how your breathing affects the separate parts and the whole of your body as air moves freely in and out of your lungs. You might want to focus on the whole body or just parts of the body, and that is OK. When you notice any tension in your body, breathe out and let the tension leave with your breath.

Step 1: Put yourself in a comfortable position that you will be able to maintain for a period of time. This can be standing up, lying down or sitting in a chair. Ensure the room is warm enough for you to stay inactive for a while and that you won't be disturbed. If you can, take your shoes off, and if you feel comfortable, shut your eyes. If any outside noise bothers you, notice this and, unless it's an emergency, let the distraction go.

Step 2: Take a few moments to clear your mind of any thought you might have; these things will still be there when you finish, and you can deal with them then.

Step 3: Once your mind is clear and you're not distracted, sit, lie or stand as still as you can. Direct your attention towards your breathing and become aware and notice the rhythm of your breath. Notice the air coming in and out of your body; don't change how you're breathing, just breathe as you are and notice that you're breathing.

Step 4: Now, direct your attention to your clothing on your body, the floor against you or the temperature of the room. Don't judge what you notice; you're just observing and finding the words to describe what you notice.

Step 5: Now, move your attention towards your body. Are any parts sore, tender or sensitive? How do your muscles feel? Does any part of your body feel light or heavy, tense or relaxed? Once you have done this, start at your toes and work up, noticing as you go your toes (on both feet); wiggle them and observe what you notice.

Next, direct your attention on to the rest of your foot. Is your sole (if standing or sitting) or your heal (if you're lying on your back) on the floor? Can you feel the texture of the ground on your feet? This is a great activity to do on grass or the beach.

Move up from your feet to your ankles. You may wish to move them, rotate them and notice the movement of the joints in addition to how this changes how your feet feel on the surface they're on.

Move up your lower legs, your shins and calves and then towards your knees and then thighs. Again, notice what you can feel, don't judge what you notice. You may wish to gently tense and relax your muscles and observe the difference in how that feels, how the muscles feel lighter after being tensed for a brief moment.

Move up from your legs to your pelvis, your buttocks and then towards your stomach. Can you notice your abdomen and chest moving as you breathe? Don't judge what you notice or if you can't notice that, just observe. Then move your attention towards your back, notice your lower and upper back, the curve of your spine; notice it against the surface you're resting upon. Move your attention towards your ribs and how they move around from your back to your front.

As your attention comes to the top of your chest, notice your shoulders, shrug and move them if you wish and notice how this feels. Direct your attention down your arms; begin at the upper arm and notice how it connects to the shoulder. Then move down to your elbow and the lower arm. If you wish, move your arms and notice what you feel, or tense and relax them and observe the change in sensation.

Then, at your wrist, let your attention move down each finger. Are they resting or touching anything; if so, what can you observe? Rotate your wrist, wiggle your fingers, clench and relax your fist and observe the changing sensations. Direct your attention up your arms again towards your shoulders and then neck.

As you move up your neck towards your chin, describe what you notice about your jaw, teeth, tongue and lips. Next, move to your nose, towards your eyes, forehead and the top and then back of your head.

Step 6: You can keep doing this until you fall asleep or until you feel relaxed and tired enough to fall asleep naturally.

Below is space for you to record any observations and reflections you have form this activity.

Breathing

(you can also use this with the mindful breathing activity)

Two types of breathing exercise have been found to help people relax. Both are very simple and effective. When doing both types of breathing, try not to think of anything while doing this, just concentrate on your breathing. To start tuning into your breathing, try the following and reflect a little on what you notice;

Breath in for as long as it takes to read this slowly.

Pause for as long as it takes to read this.

Breath out for as long as it takes to read this slowly

When people become stressed and anxious about not being able to sleep, the way they breathe might change and "action breathing" become more common. This type of breathing gets more oxygen to your lungs and brain and makes you feel more alert and awake.

Technique 1: An effective way to manage this and bring your breathing back under control is by taking a long slow breath out. To do this, take a breath in and let it out with a slow long out breath and repeat.

Technique 2: Another way of breathing is called square breathing. To do this, breath in through the nose and out the mouth while counting to 4 at each step.

- inhale for the count of four
- hold it for the count of four
- exhale for the count of four
- hold for the count of four
- REPEAT

Both methods of breathing are effective. Try both and use the method you prefer. As long as your breathing is rhythmic you should find it effective. As with all things we learn, using these breathing techniques takes time and practise to become effective. Try to practice as much as you can so that you can use these techniques effectively. This will also help you stop having thoughts about if you are doing them correctly or not.

Below is space for you to record any observations and reflections you have form this activity.

_____

_____

_____

_____

_____

_____

_____

_____

_____

_____

_____

_____

_____

_____

_____

_____

_____

_____

_____

_____

_____

Progressive muscle relaxation

(you can also use this with the mindful body scan)

Progressive muscle relaxation involves tensing and relaxing different muscles in the body for a few seconds. The aim is too gently tense each much for a short duration (approximately 10 seconds), to relax them and then progress to the next muscles. I have given an outline of how to do this, but of course, you can use a different one if you are more familiar and comfortable with the one you already know.

Before the next set of muscles is tensed, it is important to notice the difference between tense and relaxed muscles. Spend a bit longer (up to 20 seconds) noticing how your relaxed muscles feel before you tense the next set of muscles.

People can find this really difficult, especially if thoughts and emotions are spinning out of control and are beginning to overwhelm them. If this happens, it is important that you maintain your focus on your muscles. If your attention wanders, refocus on the muscles you are focusing on. Combining this with mindfulness and a body scan can be quite effective to help keep your mind from wondering,

To begin with, it might be best to practice progressive muscle relaxation in a quiet place by yourself. But as you practise these techniques and get better at them, you will be able to do them anywhere. This means they'll also work as a way of distracting yourself from causes of stress as well as by stopping the physiological aspects of stress before they build up into the vicious cycle of crisis.

- Sit in a relaxed, quiet and comfortable position and loosen any tight clothing.
- Try not to think or worry about anything. Let any thoughts just enter your mind and let them go. If it helps tell yourself, you'll worry about them in 30 minutes after you've completed the progressive relaxation exercises.
- Practice on an empty stomach.
- Take some deep breaths and try to imagine the tension flowing away as you breathe out.
- Practice twice a day for at least 20 minutes per day. This will reduce as you get more skilled and experienced in relaxation and the techniques. It is essential to overlearn how to do this so that in crisis or at times of stress you will be skilled in the art of relaxation.
- You can start with any groups of muscle but until you get skilled in it, it might be worth starting with your feet and working up.
- Remember hold tense and hold each muscle for around 10 seconds and then let it go and relax for up to 20 seconds.

Feet Tense – Hold-Relax
Do this by scrunching your toes downward.

Calves Tense – Hold-Relax

Thighs Tense – Hold-Relax

Buttocks Tense – Hold-Relax
Do this by pulling them together

Stomach Tense – Hold-Relax

Do this by sucking your stomach in and holding.

Chest Tense – Hold-Relax

Do this by taking a deep breath in, holding and letting it out slowly.

Shoulders Tense – Hold-Relax

Do this by lifting your shoulders up towards your head. Then push your shoulders back as if they were going to touch together. Give this area extra attention as it can be an area where tension builds up.

Biceps and then **Triceps** Tense – Hold-Relax

Forearms and then **Fists** Tense – Hold-Relax

Neck Tense – Hold-Relax

Do this by gently stretching the back of your head back. Give this area extra attention as it can be where tension builds up. Remember to be careful when tensing this area and to do it gently.

Jaw Tense – Hold-Relax

Do this by opening your mouth widely and stretching the muscles.

Eyes Tense – Hold-Relax

Do this by closing your eyes shut.

Forehead Tense – Hold-Relax

Do this by lifting your eyebrows as high as you can.

All of this should last between 20 and 30 minutes. As you get better and your body learns how to relax, it will be quicker and more effective at relaxing.

Some people have specific routines which they do when they are at work or in public which they use as ways of controlling stress and tension in stressful situations. Once you have mastered the techniques, you can develop your own individualised relaxation programme to suit your needs. You can also use professionally made recordings and instructions of similar progressive muscle-relaxation exercises.

Below is space for you to record any observations and reflections you have form this activity.

Guided imagery

(you can also use this as a mindfulness exercise)

Guided imagery is a very effective way to calm our mind and body. Below is a brief example of a guided imagery script, if you are more familiar and comfortable with the one you already know you can, of course, use that. The example is of a beach, but you can create any version you wish, such as a woodland, or mountain. If you have a favourite place, you can use this as the focus of your imagery.

- Sit or lie in a comfortable position and relax your body, gently releasing any tension you feel.
- Starting with the top of your body allow your arms and shoulders to relax and loosen. Let the relaxation flow across your shoulders to your neck and then down your spine.
- Let the muscles from your head, down your neck, down your spine, along each of the vertebrae to relax and loosen.
- As you do so, breathe in deeply drawing air fully into your lungs. Then with a longer slower breath, breathe out and release the air. Repeat this and notice now with each breath you become more and more relaxed, letting your body become more relaxed, calm and peaceful.
- If any thoughts or emotions come to mind, other than what you are doing, notice them and let them go.
- Feel the wave of relaxation flow from the top of your head to the bottom of your feet. Notice as the wave of relaxation, flows down your spine, to your hips, down the pelvic area, to your legs, ankles and feet.

- Keeping your breathing rhythmic and smooth, spend a few moments noticing the relaxation in your feet and them allow it to flow back up your lower, then upper legs, back through your pelvic area and hips to your stomach and up through your abdomen to your chest.

- Allow your whole body to relax and rest upon the surface you are sitting or lying upon. Again, if any thoughts or emotions, other than what you are doing, or urge to do something comes to mind, notice this and let it go.

- Once your body is fully relaxed, allow the visualisation to begin.

- Imagine you are on the beach, and walking toward the sea (or walking through the woodlands or the other place you have identified)

- Notice the sound of the waves, the feel of the sand on your feet and the warmth of the sun on your face. As you observe the wind, notice the smell the sea in the air.

- In your mind continue walking along the beach towards the sea, notice the soft, warm sand underfoot and the texture you can feel. As you walk closer to the sea notice as the sand gets wetter and firmer under your feet and the foam from the wave bubbles around your toes.

- Pause and look along the beach, its wide-open expanse with the waves gently rolling in, going back and forth along the shore. Take time to savour and enjoy the repeating rhythm of the waves coming back and forth.

- Listen to the sounds of the waves, lapping along the beach and the smell of the salt water in the air.

- Notice the sun reflecting upon the water, glistening and glimmering, the bright blue of the sea with white crested waves.

- Walk along the beach, parallel to the sea, notice ocean spray upon you, the slight taste of salt in the air. The firm wet sand underfoot and the water around your toes coming back and forth in waves.

- As you walk, notice the cold water upon your feet and the warm sun upon your body. The water is clean and clear, the air fresh and invigorating. The temperature is just right, warm relaxing, soothing. Keep walking for as long as you like; you may wish to enter the water and swim and feel the sea against you or observe the birds flying above you.

- Savour and enjoy the experience; there are no worries, no stress, if any unwanted thoughts or emotions appear, notice them and let them go. Think about how calm relaxed and refreshed you feel. You have no cares, worries or woes. You are peaceful and undisturbed, resting and taking a break from the world and the hustle and bustle of daily life. Your focus and attention are upon the beach, the sea, the sounds, the smell, the taste of salt in the air, the sound of birds up above you.

- You can do this until you fall asleep or until you feel relaxed and tired enough to sleep. You don't have to just use this technique to help you sleep, you can return to this location of your guided imagery anytime you wish in the future. You can also use guided imagery during the day to give yourself a respite from any powerful thoughts, overwhelming emotions or unpleasant body sensation that you might experience and to stop you reacting mindlessly to such experiences.

Below is space for you to record any observations and reflections you have form this activity.

_____

_____

_____

_____

_____

_____

_____

_____

_____

_____

_____

_____

_____

_____

_____

_____

_____

_____

_____

Aromatherapy

(you can also use this with your mindfulness practice)

Aromas are powerful ways that memories and emotions can be evoked. This is because the olfactory nerve that gives us our sense of smell is connected to the limbic system and amygdala of our brain. This part of the brain deals with emotions, and the flight-flight-freeze-appease response. Because of this, aromas can be used as an effective way to reduce emotional agitation and relax our bodies.

For example, some studies have found that Lavender oil and Bergamot oil can calm the nervous system, may help us become more relaxed, reducing the feelings of stress and tension and be an aid to sleep.

If you are going to use essential oils to help you sleep, or for any other reason, it is advisable that you seek professional advice and follow the instructions on any product you use. Essential oils can be harmful if used in ways that were not intended to be used.

The quality of essential oils can vary widely depending upon brand and price. Always check that the brand and quality of the oil or product you use is of suitable quality and purity.

Below is space for you to record any observations and reflections you
have form this activity.

YOUR PERSONAL SLEEP IMPROVEMENT PLAN

SUMMARY CARD

Here is one-page summary that you can use to keep close by as your wellbeing and happiness crib sheet.

Sleep, Diet, Routine, Exercise

Sleep

Comfortable bed, dark and cool room, don't use blue light devices or TV in bedroom. Have a bedtime routine and get up and go to bed at the same time each day (even weekends)

When in bed use breathing techniques (square breathing in for 4, hold for 4, out for 4 or in for 4, hold for seven, then out for 8) repeat these three times and practice it through the day so you become good at it. Try this up to 8 times before bed

Be mindful of wondering and wandering mind and let go of distractions

Relax your body by tensing and relaxing

- While inhaling, focus on one muscle group and contract your muscles for 5 seconds to 10 seconds, then exhale and release the tension in that muscle group.
- Pause for 10 to 20 seconds and relax, before you move on to the next muscle group.
- Start with your toes and work your way up

How you spend your day is also important, being physically active, having a routine and eating well is also an important part of getting a good night sleep. Avoid napping during the day and using your bedroom for things other than sleeping. Try not to watch exciting films or cliff hanger series before bed as the excitement and suspense will keep you awake.

Guided imagery

In your mind think about how warm and comfortable you are feeling, how your eyelids are feeling heavy and you are able to lie comfortably in your bed and drift off to sleep. Notice your breathing and the movement in your chest and stomach of the breath coming and going as you feel sleepier and sleepier.

Thoughts

If your mind is still racing, think in as much detail about something pleasant that happened today, or what the garden looked like – I design my dream house – which provide a non-stressful alternative to focus on and help you turn away from your racing thoughts.

If after you have tried all these, get up take some deep breathes; do not turn on any bright lights or technology. Spend a few moments focusing on your breathing and being mindful. After about five minutes return to bedand start the sleep routine again.

Diet
Eat a healthy and balanced diet
Avoid processed ready meals and take always
Remember to stay hydrated throughout the day
and avoid too much caffeine and alcohol.

Routine
Have a consistent routine that makes life more predictable and hassle free
Prepare for things in advance and don't leave things to the last minutes (like ironing a shirt for work, or making your lunch)
Leave for journeys with plenty of time so you do not have to rush or stress about being late

Exercise
Being physically active is a good way to manage stress and anxiety as well as make you feel good
Being active also helps give you and appetite and get a good night sleep
You don't have to always go to the gym, you can be more active by taking the stairs instead of the lift, parking a bit further away in a car park so you have to walk a little father.
Cleaning the house, going for a walk, dancing all count as exercise

www.ingramcontent.com/pod-product-compliance
Lightning Source LLC
Chambersburg PA
CBHW020331290526
45785CB00007B/3010